The Ultimate Guide
to
Excellent Dental Care

Dr. Andrew Dine, D.D.S

General Dentist

The views and opinions reflected herein are those solely of Dr. Andrew Dine and not necessarily shared by other dentists, dental practices, dental organizations or associations. They are intended only for the purposes of information. Dr. Dine, his employees, affiliates and/or associates cannot be held liable or responsible for the information contained. Every measure possible has been taken to reference sources used in the writing of this book.

Copyright © 2017 Andrew Dine, D.D.S.

Cover designed by Ron Sheetz
Art courtesy of Shutterstock

All rights reserved.

No part of this book may be used or reproduced in any manner whatsoever without written permission of the author

Printed in the United States of America

ISBN:1542408962
ISBN-13:9781542408967

Dr. Andrew Dine, D.D.S.
12151 Nilles Rd. #16
Fairfield, OH 45014
(513) 829-9700

CONTENTS

1	My Story	7
2	Dentistry Has Been Amazon'ed	13
3	The Difficult, Grueling, Dreadful, Painful, Tiring and Unavoidable Chore of Finding Your Dentist	21
4	Delegation versus Handing Over Responsibility	27
5	The White Knuckle Flier Patient	31
6	Dental Technology - Is It As Important As Everyone Makes It Out To Be?	37
7	Dentists and Dentistry in Southwest Ohio	41
8	Brushing and Flossing	47
9	The Miracle Dental Solution	53
10	The Dreaded Cost of Dentistry It's Really Not As Bad As You Think	63
11	Treating Patients	71
12	Your Journey	89

Chapter 1 - My Story

"There is only one road to human greatness, through the school of hard knocks." Albert Einstein

---

I have been a dentist now for more than 40 years. I've seen a lot, learned a lot and experienced a lot in that time. To say dentistry has changed over the years may be an understatement and a cliché. It's an understatement in that when I first went to dental school most students graduating entered practice with a mentor, a family member or hung their own shingle out and opened a practice from the ground up. Any of these would produce excellent doctors. With the first two the doctor had the opportunity to mentor with an experienced dentist, and the last they learned under fire, or as Mr. Einstein eludes to as 'the school of hard knocks'. In any event, the doctor developed excellent skills, not only as a doctor, but also as a compassionate practitioner. The old joke in medicine is, "that's why it's called a practice".

Today, many graduating from dental school take none of these routes to practice. The dental landscape, or path to a practice is with a group practice or one managed by a dental management organization or D.M.O. There are still those that leave dental school and go into practice with their father or mother, who become their mentor. Or, they graduate and purchase an existing practice. The challenge, from my perspective, as a 40+ year dentist, many of our young graduates forego the 'mentor' path because they're eager to start making money. Because everyone knows (falsely) that dentists make a lot of money.

There are significant advantages for a new dentist to want to enter a practice or corporately managed practice. They can start making money, but do they really have the patient's best interest at heart? Now, you will likely discover as you read this book I'm a bit of a cynic. I also have a bit of an off-handed sense of humor. I tell you this because you'll have more of an opportunity to get to know me through the chapters of this book. You see, I entered dentistry because I wanted to help people. From the time I graduated from dental school I've wanted to help people get to a healthy mouth. Yes, I want to earn a good living for myself and my family, though I can do that while I also remain committed to those who commit to me... my patients. It's been my foundational philosophy from the beginning, and it remains so today.

So, why have I written this book? I started out telling you a little about how dentistry has changed since I entered practice and I did so to give you a brief perspective of what you'll find as you research dentists and dental practices in your pursuit of finding your ideal dentist. That may sound a little odd, 'Ideal dentist'. It shouldn't. Regardless of your past experiences with dentists, or even what you may have been told from others, there are some great dentists at your service. You only need to work harder at finding them. There are more dentists than any time in my history. Here's the most important piece of advice I could impart to you:

"Never **_SETTLE_** for substandard dentistry."

Remember, you're the patient. You're the one who pays the fees for care and/or treatment. You're responsible for finding the right dentist, and then, sharing in the kind of care you receive. So do your research carefully.

This is why I've written this book for you. So that you can

enter into a relationship with a dentist with your eyes wide open. As your research will find a lot of information and you will be faced with a decision to make; one you should make wisely. Those that make this decision well generally don't have to find another dentist for quite some time. Now, with that said, I'll go on record right here in saying that I'm not right for every patient. I want to be completely transparent with you. You may have had a dentist talk down to you or speak in technical terms. I will not make your feel guilty, lecture or embarrass you. I don't judge you, I want to help you.

As you'll read from several patient's comments I've included throughout this book I run a no-shame, no-guilt practice. I understand life happens and things get in the way of taking care of your teeth and it's not my place to judge... I'm not your parent, I'm your dentist. My role in our relationship is to advise and make things better. You're an adult. You can choose to do it or not.

I think before you delve deeper into this book, it would be helpful to know a little more about me as a dentist.

The Resume

I graduated from the University of Cincinnati in 1971 with a Bachelor of Science degree and then from Case Western Reserve University School of Dentistry in Cleveland, Ohio, in 1976. I chose the entrepreneurial path straight out of college and opened my own practice and have built it from the start right here in Fairfield, Ohio. I realize, reading this book, you may or may not be in my geography of the world, however, if you are, I've been serving patients in Fairfield, West Chester, Liberty Township, Fairfield Township, Middletown, Ross, Hamilton, and surrounding communities here in Butler County, Ohio.

I am a Fellow of the Academy of General Dentistry. This simply means I'm committed to continually staying educated on the advancements and changes in dentistry, in order to deliver greater care to my patients. The Fellowship is one of the most rigorous continual dental education programs a dentist can follow. It means I have advanced dental knowledge and my 40 years are the experience I've amassed in putting that knowledge to work for my patients.

I also have advanced training and experience with Invisalign, the latest and one of the most proficient orthodontic teeth alignment systems available for patients.

I'm also a member of the American Dental Association, Ohio Dental Association, Cincinnati Dental Society, and Academy of General Dentistry. My practice also is a member of the Better Business Bureau.

I've chosen dentistry as my profession, as stated earlier, because I can help people improve their lives on a daily basis. It gives me great satisfaction to see the amazing improvements I'm able to make in people's oral health because, a healthy mouth leads to a healthy body, I know the work that I do does a lot of good for a lot of people.

People come to me for their own specific reason, such as being in pain or wanting to keep their teeth for their entire life. My dental philosophy is that the basic end result I want, for you, is a healthy mouth for your entire life. If that's what you want too, and you're in my area, we should meet because we can accomplish great things for you, together.

I don't push patients into doing anything they don't need or want. I do however, I present every patient with the facts of their mouth and options for fixing the problems. If that means presenting treatment options then that's what I'll do. I'm not a salesmen peddling a used car to a non-buyer. Doctor's are not salesmen regardless of what you may think. You may have had that experience at your last dentist, but you won't experience it here. With that said however, don't take offense when your dentist (even I) presents you with a treatment plan. Yes it'll be the last thing you'll want to hear when you come in for an exam, cleaning or check up, but it's my duty as a professional doctor to present you the facts. Were I a heart surgeon you would not want me to hide the fact that you may be facing a heart attack if you didn't get treatment. Fortunately for me (and you) most dental procedures aren't as life threatening as a those of the heart.

Tooth decay and gum disease are totally preventable, so you should be able to keep your teeth your entire life.

If you find, as you read this book, I sound like the kind of dentist you'd like taking care of you, then I'd welcome the opportunity. You will find information about scheduling an appointment with me in Chapter 12. If you're not in my 'neck of the woods', or you find you don't like me, that's okay too. I know you'll find this book to be helpful in navigating the shark infested waters of finding a dentist for you and your family.

Thank you for picking my book, more importantly, picking it up, cracking the cover and starting to read it. You're now on the right path to finding your ideal dentist.

Remember, never settle for substandard dentistry!

The primary reason I was compelled to write this book was to help more people find their 'right' dentist. I define 'right' as one who will listen to your dental concerns and problems, understand them and be compassionate in offering advice and solutions. Too often we as dentists get the bad rap as peddling unnecessary dentistry. There are charlatans in the field who do that, but for the most part, there are a lot of good dentists to be found. This book will prepare you with the information and education you need to measure, judge and determine if a dentist is right for you.

Good hunting!

Chapter 2 - Dentistry Has Been Amazon'ed

"It is our choices, Harry, that show what we truly are, far more than our abilities." J.K. Rowling - Harry Potter and the Chamber of Secrets

---

I think by now virtually everyone on the planet is familiar with who and what Amazon is. If you're one of those few who may be living like a hermit and are completely disconnected from the digital world I'll provide a brief description of Amazon.

In the big broad picture of it, Amazon is an international digital commerce company. Originally an online bookstore (physical books). Today Amazon offers a wide variety of physical (and digital) products and the reach of their category offerings is continuing to expand. Today they are the largest internet-based retailer in the world. Now that's important to know because on their current course of expansion, I would predict, they will ultimately enter the dental practice market. That could be good and it could be bad, but it's not my objective here to pass judgment on that.

However, if you're not aware, there are large companies who've beat Amazon to the dental field. These companies are known as Dental Support Organizations.
(https://en.wikipedia.org/wiki/Dental_Service_Organizations)

You're always faced with balancing the cost of dentistry and your budget. Dental insurance, unlike medical insurance has limitations based on the plan. Deductibles and maximum limits vary, and renew annually. It would be much easier to get the kind of dental care you'd like if dental insurance were the same as medical insurance, but it's not. Unfortunately that's the reality we have to live with. I do everything I can to help the patient balance this. Later I talk about the dreaded costs of dentistry (Chapter 10), though here I think its important to put into perspective how you view the 'cost' of dentistry.

I titled this chapter "Dentistry Has Been Amazon'ed" to make a point that more and more products and services are becoming more easily available to us. Amazon has made it easier to buy books and other products online, saving us time and in many cases money. This convenience is good, and saving money is always good, but in creating time and money savings Amazon has commoditized a great many things that weren't before. In the process that commoditizing diminishes the value. Which leads me to what I think is important to consider when you're searching for a dentists and/or dental care.

A great many things can be valued based on their price. Books for example. J.K. Rowling's Harry Potter books are the same regardless of where you purchase them. You can buy them from Amazon and pay less than you would at the local Barnes and Noble book store. The book is the same it's just the price that's different. That would be smart price shopping, but not all things can be valued by their price or fee. Dentistry is one of those things you shouldn't make a decision based entirely on fees. You can see two different dentists and receive two different levels of care and quality of their work. They both know dentistry, but how they approach your treatment and care may be drastically different. You may pay the same fee for both, but you may find one more caring and pain free than the other.

Additionally, you buy a book, but invest in dentistry. Dentistry, even cleanings and exams is something more impactful on you than reading a good book. You can hate the book, but when you're finished you're done with it. A bad experience at the dentists sticks with you. If you don't believe me ask someone who had a bad experience as a child and today breaks out into a cold sweat at the thought of going to a dentist.

I believe that most people would agree the most important factors in their dental cost would be:

- The experience (how they're treated)
- The level and quality of care (the dentist's skill)
- The fee (or price)

So, here's a formula I'd suggest in deciding on the value of what a dentist may provide, based on his or her fees. To do so I'll use an auto repair example. As a dentist I'm a service provider. An auto mechanic is a service provider. I fix problems in your mouth and the auto mechanic fixes problems with your car.

There are three criteria to use in measuring (dentists or auto mechanics)

1. Price
2. Quality
3. Service

I call this the pick two principle. Of these three criteria you can only ever get two of them. For example, if you decide that price and quality is most important to you, you sacrifice service. If quality and service are most important then you'll likely pay a higher price in order to get the quality and service.

Here's the principle applied to auto repair.

Let's say your car breaks down, specifically your transmission. I picked the transmission because it's a fundamental component of your vehicle. You're car can't take you anywhere, you can't take the kids to soccer practice or meet your friend for coffee if your transmission doesn't work. So what do you do if you don't have a regular, trusted auto mechanic? You probably go online and search 'transmission auto repair' in Grandpa Google. At the time of writing this book I found 50,800 results in Google for 'transmission auto repair Fairfield Ohio, or 351,000 results for a more general 'auto repair Fairfield Ohio'. Let's consider the former of the two. Wow! Over 50,000 results. Sure, you're not going to go through all of those, but you're at least going to start at the top of the page and work your way down.

The first 6 results were actual shops in town. Arbitrarily pick 3 of them and call and ask, "How much would it cost to fix my transmission?" I understand that's a very broad question. Make, model and the year of your car will matter, but let's consider all things are equal, remember, this is for demonstration purposes.

Like any reasonable adult you're looking for the least expensive option, because you know it's probably going to be expensive. How can't it be, it's a transmission. So initially you're looking for a price to be quoted to you over the phone. The first shop says it'll be $2,250. The second shop says it'll be $3,500 and the third $5,000. Based entirely on price you decide to go with the quote from the first shop because it's the cheapest. You take your car in and have the work done. Upon completion you pay your money and 6 months later the transmission starts leaking fluid all over the engine and smoke starts to billow out from under your hood. You call the shop that replaced the transmission and they say "sorry, there's nothing we can do". In this situation you selected the shop based on their price and you received an equal level of quality... poor. Little did you know the transmission the shop installed was found in a similar car as yours at a junk yard. They simply pulled it from the wreck, cleaned it up, put it in your car, filled it with fluid and sent you on your way. You got price and quality (low quality albeit), but you sacrificed service.

Second scenario, you select the shop that quoted you the middle price, $3,500 and the same situation happens after the service, you have a problem with the transmission. With paying a little more the shop provided a warranty on the transmission so you don't have to pay for a replacement or service on that unit. They're able to give you a warranty because the transmission is a rebuilt unit and they can provide a warranty on it. You however do have to pay for the service work the shop performs, but the part or parts are warranted. You got price (though a little higher because the transmission was rebuilt and cost a little more) and you received service because they could afford to offer you a warranty. You didn't however get the best quality repair because of a lesser quality part.

Now, consider had you chosen the higher priced service option at $5,000. Again, transmission problems happen 6 months after the replacement. You call the shop and to your surprise they replace or repair the transmission and your bill for the work is $0. The part was remanufactured (by the manufacturer) so it was warranted 100% and you weren't charged any labor or service fees because the shop is reputable and they calculate in such conditions in their fees. You got the best quality and the highest service, but you sacrificed a cheap price.

The point is that your view of price will be completely different after you've received the service. You've heard the saying, *"You get what you pay for"*. Price is what you pay, but value is what you get. The same holds true in dentistry. Fundamentally all dentists are alike. We've all graduated dental school with similar credentials. Just as there were three factors in my transmission example, there also are three value factors you must take into consideration when choosing a dentist. They are skill, experience and personality. Often, a dentist's personality or the quality of their people skills, or how well they treat patients, is referred to as their 'chairside manner', much like a physician's bedside manner.

These three factors are even more measurable than are price, quality and service. Skill and experience is something every dentist possesses in differing degrees, but chairside manners can vary greatly. For many patients, these factors are the most critical when choosing a dentist. Unlike my fee, quality and service example, with dentists you do get all three factors of skill, experience and chairside manner, this varies from dentist to dentist. You have a lot of choices when it comes to who you choose as your dentist, so choose wisely. And that will be the subject for my next chapter.

A patient's perspective: *"I was scared of the dentist"* - John Halase

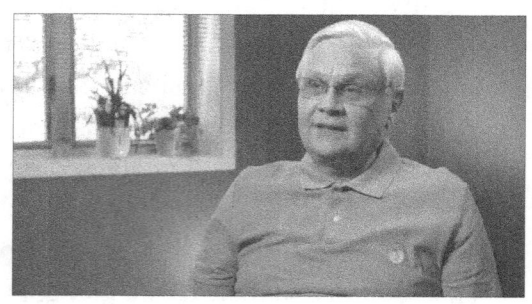

"I was a person that was afraid of needles. I did not like to get vaccinations or anything. Sometimes when a procedure is going on, Dr. Dine will check with you, do you feel that – it's continually through whatever he's doing with you, he's assuring that you're not feeling any discomfort.

The fear of going to the dentist sometimes gets started when you're a child, and if your first experience with a dentist is somebody that doesn't care, that kind of sets into your mind, into your adulthood.

Like I said, we were very fortunate with Dr. Dine, from the beginning, it was a positive impression.

A lot of times when you come to a dentist office, you're nervous. It's not something that people look forward to doing. But when you come to Dr. Dine's office, they make you feel more relaxed. From the time that you sign in, to the experience, whether they are cleaning your teeth or doing something more than that. Fortunately, because like I said, over 30 years that I have been with Dr. Dine, we have this regular thing where he makes sure my teeth are in good health. I don't have the problems maybe somebody might have if they don't have a doctor they go to regularly.

Whenever I recommend people, I take my word as something that I hold valuable, so I don't just recommend anybody. My sister in law comes to him. I've recommended family and friends. People that I know I am going to see again, I recommend to Dr. Dine."

I am accepting new patients. You can schedule an appointment by calling (513) 829-9700 or visiting www.DrDine.com to request an appointment online.

Dr. Andrew Dine

Chapter 3: The Difficult, Grueling, Dreadful, Painful, Tiring & Unavoidable Chore of Finding Your Dentist

"The harder thing to do and the right thing to do are usually the same thing." Author - Unknown

---

In my grandparents day you picked a dentist based on who you knew, or felt comfortable with. Often times your dentist was a family friend or a familiar face in the community. Really not much has changed about it today. Yes the Internet has made it more confusing. There's a lot of free information about dentists, dental practices and dentistry available at your fingertips, with the stroke of a few keys on your keyboard, but really what does all that tell you?

I'm reminded of a friend who's mother was in the market for a new vehicle. Her current van was getting up there in miles and the repairs were starting to become more frequent and more expensive and she'd finally made up her mind it was time to replace it rather than continue to sink good money after more good money into repairs. After she decided between two makes of cars she began to narrow in on specifically what model car between those two manufacturers. Then she went online and started doing her due diligence. She looked at safety ratings, gas mileage, average cost to operate the car annually, average cost of repairs, etc, etc.

After about 2 months of exhaustive research she was armed with a mountain of information. She even went as far as to talk with service stations and ask their opinion which cars were more reliable from a maintenance standpoint. From them she got entirely new information. Some supported the research she'd gathered and others were contradictive to what she'd found. After two months of this her current vehicle needed repairs yet again. Now she was faced with the do or die situation. Should she sink a little more money into repairs or bite the bullet and go for the new car, but which car? She called her son to ask his opinion and after she'd told him of all the data and material she'd gathered, spent hours and hours of time pouring over the research, her son asked her a simple question, "Mom, after doing all this research are you more informed or more confused?" She thought for a moment and then exclaimed in desperation, "More confused!"

What her son said next was so simple but revolutionary. He asked her, "What does your gut tell you?" That revealed her answer. The same is true when you're looking for a dentist. In my grandparent's time they relied more on instinct than on information, because they didn't have the abundance of information we have available today. What does your gut tell you about a dentist.

Don't get me wrong, you <u>should</u> do your due diligence and research on dentists. Having dental work done, even regular checkups and cleanings is not something you should take lightly. Despite many big businesses and DSO organization's attempts at making dental treatment more like buying toilet paper, you are the one who pays for, and has to live with the results of treatment. It's much like the story of ham and eggs. The chicken can lay an egg and walk away, but the pig is there to stay. Dental care is not something one should make a decision on trivially.

Many of my patients come to me from referrals. An existing patient will refer a friend, family member or coworker. In my grandparent's day it was the most valuable way to judge a dentist's skill, experience and character. Just as I described in the previous chapter, no two dentists are created equally. The deciding factor on most dentists for patients comes down to how that dentist makes them feel as a patient. Unfortunately there are a lot of patients who continue with a dentist whom they are uncomfortable, but continue because the thought of finding a new one is more painful a task than enduring the existing one. They fear the 'out of the frying pan and into the fire' syndrome. They're afraid they may go from a not so good dentist to an even worse dentist. This is where your due diligence and taking the advice of others about a dentist can be your most valuable research. If you don't know people who have experience with a particular dentist, then search out what others say about him or her.

Yes, most dentists have a website, but I go so far as to provide you with as much transparent information about me, and my practice, in advance of visiting my practice for the first time. Any dentist who's been in practice as long as I have (40+ years) should be able to anticipate the questions and concerns you have about seeing the dentist. For just such a thing I created a DVD where I answer a lot of those common questions and concerns. Questions like, "I don't like the shots, will it hurt in your practice?" "What about insurance?" to name a few. On that DVD you also will hear patients tell their stories of fear and anxiety of going to a dentist.

Choosing a dentist should be something you only do once, if you chose wisely. It doesn't have to be difficult. My advice is simple. I said it before, but it's worth restating, do your research, listen to people who have experience with the dentist and then do as my friend's mom did in choosing a car, narrow it down to two dentists, then trust your gut, listen to your instincts as to which is right for you. The human instinct has been with us for more than 6 million years and it has served us pretty well in that time, I think yours will serve you pretty well too.

A patient's perspective: *"I used to avoid the dental office at all costs"* - Tashenna Baker

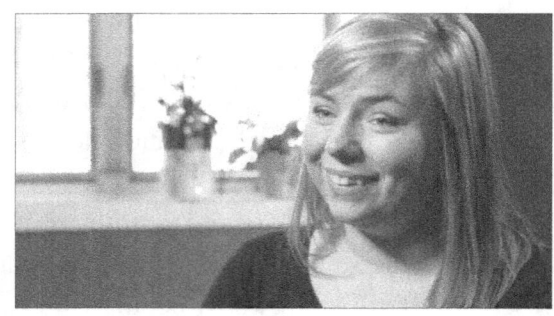

" I used to dread going to the dentist. I would think about it, I would schedule the appointment three weeks before and I would be shaking about it before we were even close. But now, I come here, it's quick and I forget it's even the dentist really. It's a different ball game. It's completely different.

When I first came in, I'm horrified of the shots that they give you, and everything. I was shaking, I was so scared. The very first impression I had, he put a vibrating stick, I don't know what the tool is called, but he put it on my gums to help numb where the shot went in. And then they gave me the gas, but before doing that they calmed everything. It was really serene, and I'm pretty sure I fell asleep while getting it done. It was great, it was wonderful actually.

This office is very prompt. I'm so accustomed to going to dentists where you sit for thirty minutes before getting in but they're very quick to get your paperwork to you, get it filled out and then you get back in ten minutes and you're out twenty-five minutes later. Regardless, I was concerned at first because I had allotted an hour and a half for a cleaning and I saw that there was several other patients. Only Dr. Dine was here and it was still twenty minutes and I was out. It was great.

They said he was painless and he was really nice and calming, and I have anxiety so terribly so; he was out of my network still but the prices were comparable so I just came here anyways and loved it. Now I get everyone to come here, they're annoyed with me. I'm just like, you have to try him, I promise you're going to love it. Always, I'm just so excited about this place."

If you'd like to receive a copy of the DVD companion to this book, call my office at (513) 829-9700. I am accepting new patients. You can schedule an appointment by calling (513) 829-9700 or visiting www.DrDine.com to request an appointment online.

Dr. Andrew Dine

Chapter 4 - Delegation vs. Handing Over Responsibility

"The problem with communication is the illusion that it has taken place."
Leonard Bernard Shaw - Irish Playwright

Trust is a foundational principle in the relationship between a dentist and his or her patient. Responsibility and communication are another two principles critical to the successful relationship between the doctor and those in his or her care.

As a patient you seek out a general dentist to diagnose and care for your overall oral health. There are a number of things you automatically assume the dentist possesses. You would expect he or she is a licensed professional. Because they have an office and the name on the door is preceded by Dr. or followed by D.D.S. you automatically expect they've completed the necessary study to get the qualifications... and you'd be correct.

> **Dentistry** is a branch of medicine that is involved in the study, diagnosis, prevention, and treatment of diseases, disorders and conditions of the oral cavity (mouth).

You expect the person you see for your oral health to have a certain set of professional skills and training. You expect them to be knowledgeable on the science of dentistry and the human mouth, keep up on the latest technologies as they pertain to the duties of administering great oral health care and provide you with the best and least intrusive care possible...meaning they won't inflict pain upon you physically, emotionally or psychologically. In short that's what you'd expect from a professional dentist; or at least should expect.

Historically, the relationship between the dentist and patient was often one-sided, meaning the dentist diagnosed and dictated treatment and the patient accepted what the doctor prescribed, without questions. Sounds crazy right? That's how the relationship looked 100 years ago, but it doesn't today. On the other hand, 100 years ago it wasn't uncommon for the dentist to be invited out to your home for the check up or treatment.

The relationship with your dentist has changed from what it once was. The diagnosis is largely on the part of the dentist, but today the decision of treatment and care is shared between you and your dentist, as it should be. Shared decision making on your treatment is more the standard today, but there are dentists who wouldn't share this position. It's important you be aware of the dentist you seek as to their opinion on how the recommended treatment should be discussed and decided on.

As a patient you delegate your responsibility to the dentist to examine and make a diagnosis of what he or she finds from an exam. Often the conversation about potential treatment starts with the hygienists, when you're in for a biannual or routine cleaning. The hygienist may identify something out of the ordinary and communicate it to the dentist. The dentist will then investigate further to see if there is an issue present, something that needs to be addressed.

However, there is a lot more to dental care and your experience with it. Never lose sight of this. You're an adult. You have the right to chose the kind of dental care and experience you want. You don't have to settle.

Remember when you were a child and you didn't know how things were, you created things your way, you made believe and in that make believe things were reality, your reality. When we grow up though and become adults we're shown things the way they are and told they are what they are, and that we should accept them, and we do. In that acceptance though we accept things we wouldn't have, shouldn't have, because deep down we know they weren't right, but it's easier to accept things the way they are because questioning it is too difficult, too controversial. The reality though is, as adults, and as American's you have the right to question and choose. No one should ever accept anything substandard, especially in something that can have a significant effect on one's health. It is for this reason that a patient and dentist today share in their care and treatment. It once wasn't that way, but it is today and you have the right to it, to excellent dental care, from a dentist you're comfortable with, one you like and most importantly you trust.

You're not the dentist. You don't have the specialized training, but you do know yourself. Because of it you do have to delegate your care to one you trust. You will know the right dentist when you find him or her. But you should never hand over responsibility for your health and that of your family. It is my responsibility as a dentist to care for my patients following the absolute best course that is right for them, but in order to do that the patient, you, has to participate in the care 100%.

Dentistry, unlike other medical professions has kept its roots in the family tradition. In its earliest existence dentists were trusted advisors and friends. Not much has changed today. When you find a dentist and a practice that maintains this 'family-like' tradition you'll know it when you see it. You'll hear it from patients, and very often those patients will have been with that dentist for a long time.

In closing out this chapter my message is simple, never hand over responsibility for your care, rather find a dentist in whom you can partner with.

A patient's perspective: *"Dr. Dine personally calls after a procedure to check on me "* - **John Crowley**

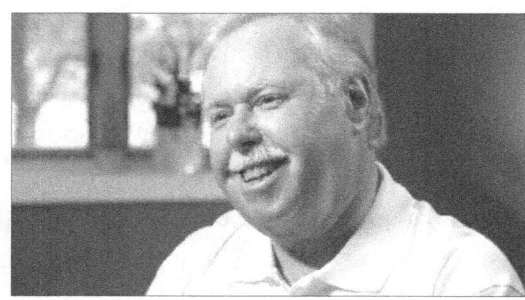

" I guess when I was young, I had some stuff done and it was painful, and when I got older and I didn't have to go, I did as little as possible. It caught up with me, and he needed to help straighten me out; which he did. I'm a regular, I'm here every few months.

Basically, Dr. Dine has been – I've been to a dentist before here I got here, but it was in and out and another guy here and there – but once I came to him, I haven't changed. Like I said, we've got a good relationship. He's friendly, always happy to see you, glad that you came, and he makes it as painless as possible. That's a good thing; it keeps you coming back.

Dr. Dine is very personable because he remembers you. He remembers the history, he remembers what you do for a living, he remembers some of the obstacles that you have to deal with just to get here and he's very good at working around my schedule. One other thing is, if you had a procedure done, he personally would call you after that and say, hey is everything okay, are you feeling alright; which I never had happen before so that was kind of nice. It's a nice little place to come into. They hustle and bustle, you get in, you get what you want done and you get out."

I am accepting new patients. You can schedule an appointment by calling (513) 829-9700 or visiting www.DrDine.com to request an appointment online.

Chapter 5 - The White Knuckle Flier Patient

"The truth of the matter is that you always know the right thing to do. The hard part is doing it." General Norman Schwarzkopf

---

There is dental anxiety and then there is dental phobia. More than 74% of the US population has dental anxiety. Anxiety is not looking forward to going to the dentist. It's a universal phenomenon so don't feel anxious about being anxious. Nearly 223 million others in America feel the same as you may. Merriam-Webster's dictionary defines anxiety as:

> anx-i-ety *n.* 1 a: painful or apprehensive uneasiness of mind over an impending or anticipated ill b: fearful concern or interest c: a cause of anxiety 2: an abnormal and overwhelming sense of apprehension and fear often marked by physiological signs, by doubt concerning the reality and nature of the threat, and by self-doubt about one's capacity to cope with it.

Simplified, the anxiety is real, though experienced emotionally, which triggers the physical response of fear. It's a simple and clear definition of what one experiences, but not something to take lightly. However, you can rest assured you're not alone.

In contrast there's dental phobia, which is more severe. Virtually 9%-12% of the US population has a phobia against going to the dentist. Again, for clarity, the definition of phobia according to Merriman-Webster:

> pho-bia *n.* an exaggerated, inexplicable and illogical fear of a particular object, class of objects or situation.

Again, simplified, a fear that isn't real, but does exist. Phobia is a heightened state of anxiety. It can leave people panic-stricken and terrified. They often know the fear is irrational (as defined), but feel helpless to do anything about it. This can often lead to years of avoiding the dentist. I have many patients who fit in both the anxiety and phobia categories. You can see and hear from many of them on my website at www.DrDine.com.

The most common cause of a patient's anxiety or phobia can be traced to a past experience. I remember my professor telling story after story of patient cases who had bad experiences with their dentists.

I remember one story about a 9 year old boy who went into the dentist for work on a back molar. The dentist failed to properly anesthetize him and when the dentist started work on the tooth he hit the nerve dead on. The professor said that patient continued going to dentists, often under duress, until he stopped all together when he became an adult. The boy said he couldn't even drive past a dentist's office without breaking out into a cold sweat.

I'm sure if you're a person who is anxious or phobic about the dentist it's probably a bit uncomfortable to read of such a case. You may have had a similar situation.

As you read from the dictionary definition about anxiety and phobia, in almost all cases the fear is either not real or it's caused by a past memory. As my professor used to say, "Good patients who experienced well intentioned dentists". The reality is that most dental visits are pain free, or they should be. A good dentist never forgets what it's like to be the patient in the chair. It may come as a surprise, but dentists go to dentists. I have a dentist I see at least twice a year. I get dental cleanings done and I've had dental work performed in my mouth. So like you, I'm a patient too, and when I see a patient I always put myself in their seat, as the patient.

I have worked with a lot of fearful, anxious and phobic patients. Many of my patients would tell you I'm very good at easing their fears and anxieties.

I have several strategies to help patients past their fears. These are part of the unique experience in my practice. They're part of what I call the Dine Method. Many years ago these used to be added benefits of a dental practice, but today they should be mandatory, yet not all practices offer these patient comfort conveniences. My patient's comfort is the first concern, before I ever start treating a patient. I have a number of comfort options available for patients. Likely the most uncomfortable part of seeing the dentists are the dreaded shots we administer. I'm with you, I don't like them either. They are however an important part of making you comfortable for treatments. So I've research far and wide to find the pain-free method of giving my patients Novocain. My DentalVibe is a painless shot. Yes, painless! I'll understand if you don't believe me. You really do have to experience it to believe me. So for now, go with me on faith.

Magicians have magic wands, I have a DentalVibe, and it's a neat tool. Actually, now that I think about it, it's my magic wand. First, it doesn't look like a typical needle, so your brain won't register it as one. Second, the tip of the DentalVibe has two soft, gentle probes that touch the surface of your gum, ever so slightly. The instant the tip touches your gum tissue, it creates a vibration that sends a signal to your brain. Within 10 seconds of transmission of that signal, the pain gates of your brain close, blocking the sensation of pain you would normally feel from a traditional shot and injection needle. My patients love it.

In addition to my DentalVibe, I also have comfortable, reclining chairs. I've actually had some patients who are so comfortable they fall asleep during cleanings and treatment. I also provide music and soft, warm comfy blankets. A lot of ladies tell me they get cold, despite us keeping the office at a comfortable temperature.

If that's not enough to ease your fears I also offer Dental Sedation. You probably know it as laughing or happy gas. Actually it's a safe nitrous oxide sedation. It has no color, no smell and it won't bother you. I've had patients tell me they feel "happy drunk" with the nitrous. It does work. It helps you relax and feel care-free before your dental treatment begins. Despite the gas being free of any odor, we do have scented masks to give patients an added level of comfort. Our happy gas is a mild sedative and can be used for almost any procedure, including dental cleanings and exams.

The most important component in making patients feel comfortable is my compassionate dental staff. Just like me, my staff are dental patients too and they understand what you are going through, and can make your time here a breeze. Whatever you need while you are with us, you simply let us know. The sign for patients who need to stop or take a break is to simply raise their hand and we stop. You raise your hand because many times you can't talk because your mouth is full. And yes, I will often talk with you when you won't be able to answer, but that's okay, I'm used to it. I can promise you though, you will never hear a lecture from me or be made to feel guilty. I'm your dentist not your parent.

A patient's perspective: *"I've been coming to Dr. Dine for over 11 years now "* - Sarilda Conover

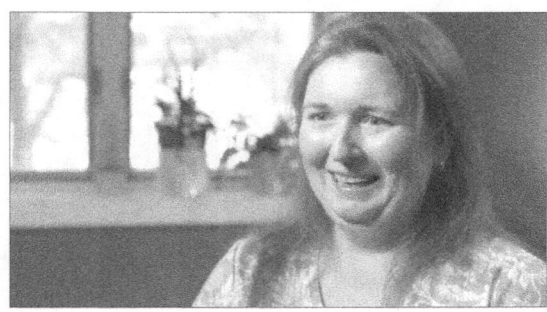

" The amount of dentists that I have been to in my life have surpassed the number of years that I've been with Dr. Dine. He has been the one dentist I've been with for more than eleven years. He is just magnificent because he is absolutely cheerful, he has never yelled at me, I've never had any anxiety coming in here.

He uses the supersonic to clear off the tartar plaque on your teeth and it's still a high sound which is uncomfortable to hear but he allows me to wear my headphones and I just crank it up. He maneuvers my mouth any which way he needs it. There was absolutely no way that any other dentist was going to make me comfortable with it as he did. The fact that he gave me gas relaxed me quite a bit and he made sure that it was good and well, affected me. The Novocain that he put in, yes it stings a little bit when he sticks the needle in to coat the area but I didn't feel anything when he did. I just did not feel anything. And even afterwards, I don't remember any pain.

If he can work wonders with me, he can work wonders with anyone. I just did not want to go to the dentist at all and I finally broke down; I had to do it. They have always gone above and beyond their duty to make sure my experience was pleasant."

I am accepting new patients. You can schedule an appointment by calling (513) 829-9700 or visiting www.DrDine.com to request an appointment online.

Dr. Andrew Dine

Chapter 6 - Dental Technology - Is It As Important As Everyone Makes It Out To Be?

"If you align expectations with reality, you will never be disappointed."

Terrell Owens

"With advances in dental technology, oral health problems can be caught and treated earlier and quicker. The solutions for oral health are more promising than they have ever been. Dentists and patients benefit from the advances in dental technology." That's what I typically hear from the sales representatives who visit my office to show the latest dental technology. That statement is accurate, though it's not the most important thing for you as a patient to be focused on when searching for the right dentist for you and your family. Your interests should be more self-centered, around you.

If you were to dissect a dental practice like an apple pie, there'd be four primary slices. Most dental practices have four identifiable areas or departments, using a corporate terminology. They would be:

1. The dentist and his or her assistant(s). These are the people you come in direct contact with for your dental care and treatment
2. Dental hygiene - The people who clean your teeth
3. The office people
4. The technology

This is an over-simplification as to the actual structure and functionality of a dental practice, though I'm simplifying for the discussion of technology in this chapter. The key point to understand is that technology is important. However, many dental practices will give technology greater importance in their marketing and advertising than they should. Here's why. Consider the four parts of the dental pie I listed. Three of the four components are people and only one is technology. My point is you'll come in contact with people more often and more frequently than you will technology. Your experience in our practice will be based more on the relationship you have with my team than it will be on the relationship you have with my technology.

Now, that may sound silly, though it's factual. For example, I have a digital x-ray machine that is unique in that it takes panoramic x-rays (360 image of your mouth), the bitewings, which traditionally you had to hold x-ray panels in your mouth and have the camera put to your cheek. It also emits 80% less radiation, is more comfortable and convenient for the patient because it's less invasive. It's a wonderful machine. Patients like it when they find out how much more comfortable and safe it is to get x-rays, but no one has ever left my office and said they loved the digital x-ray machine so much they were coming back because of it. It sounds crazy, but it's true. The technology we use in your treatment is important, though they are only tools.

You don't see an auto repair shop advertising they use wrenches to repair your car. You expect an auto mechanic to have the tools they need to perform the repairs. It is the auto mechanic's responsibility to have the tools they need to perform the work. The same holds true with your dentist. It is his or her responsibility to have the right tools to do the work. Now, advancement in dental technology progresses more rapidly than those of auto repair, so we have to constantly keep up on the latest technology, and we do. In addition to keeping up on technology we also take continuing education courses to stay up to date on the latest techniques. It's all done in the effort to make your experiences the most pleasant and pain free as possible.

With respect to my physician counterparts, I don't have to experiment as much as a physician when it comes to treatment. Unlike general medicine, dentistry is pretty exacting, it really is much more scientific. The results are more predictable and immediate than that you might experience in general medicine. I'm not suggesting a dentist's work is easier or harder than that of a physician, though they're different. Dental technology has drastically changed the way I'm able to diagnose and treat patients, though it's the personal interaction and care that is far more important than the machines and gizmos I use to treat you. My focus has always been on the patient and not on trying to impress anyone with fancy, expensive equipment.

So if you see a dentist advertising that he or she has the latest technology that money can buy you should run away from that practice as fast as you can. They should be more focused on assuring you that you'll be well cared for, not showing off their latest dental 'toys'.

Rest assured I have all the latest technologies available to me to make your care the best it can be. But understand I'm more focused on promoting how well we'll take care of you than I am trying to impress you with a bunch of expensive dental tools, most of which you would not know how to identify an old machine from a new one. My patients care that I have the latest technology, but only as it pertains to how well I can take care of them. You should too.

A patient's perspective: "Dr. Dine does everything much better than everybody else does " - David Gray

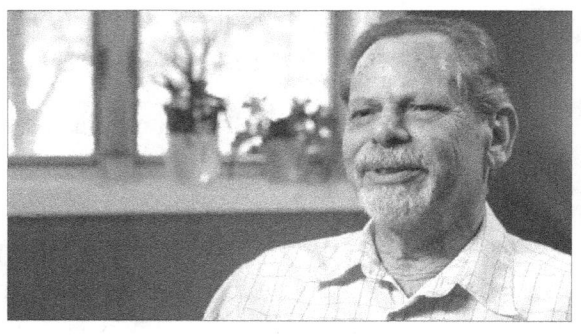

"I have two daughters in different dental practices but I keep coming back to Dr. Dine. For me, he does everything much better than everybody else does. I can get almost for free in my two daughter's places but I don't want to go there because Dr. Dine is so efficient. Every time that he works with me he checks thoroughly everything that I need; and other dentists sometimes they don't even come in and check if they have a hygienist. I don't like that feel; I like the personal attention that I get from Dr. Dine.

Some dentists don't care. They just want to get in there and get the job done. Dr. Dine is extremely efficient by the way, he doesn't waste any time. You can tell that he is extremely efficient on every tooth, every surface of your tooth, but he doesn't miss any of them all the way around, and before you can blink your eyes, he's finished because of his skill.

That's another thing I like about Dr. Dine, he keeps some updated equipment going. He likes new style, new technology of things to do. The cleanliness as far as he goes is a lot superior to a lot of the dentist offices I've been in. So I feel comfortable in coming in, knowing that he's got late technology, good equipment to work with, and his expertise is the real reason why I come in."

I am accepting new patients. You can schedule an appointment by calling (513) 829-9700 or visiting www.DrDine.com to request an appointment online.

Chapter 7: Dentists & Dentistry in Southwestern Ohio

"How do you know when you're in love?" Cupid

It's a question that is as eternal as time itself. We could debate the philosophical aspects of the question, but the key is that when you know it you know it instinctively. Instinct is a great and accurate barometer if we listen to it. You will find an abundance of data available on any subject you search, including dentists in Southwestern Ohio, where my practice is located.

Much of this book is applicable to any patient in any part of the country. This chapter however is devoted specifically to those people in my geographic area. There will, however, be some valuable information you may take away from it, if you are elsewhere in the US.

Searching for a dentist, whether a new one, because you've just moved into the area, or you're ready for a change, can be confusing and a costly one if you make the wrong choice. It can be very confusing when you start investigating the options available to you. The Internet can be wonderful for finding a restaurant for dinner. Restaurants all offer the same things, food and an experience. Their cuisine can differ based on culture and taste, but they all serve food. Fundamentally they serve a basic need. You can pick a restaurant online, visit it, pay your money and have a bad meal, but when it's over, it's over. Finding the right dentist for you and your family is much more complicated. The ramifications from the decision about a restaurant and a poor meal will soon be forgotten, but the decision about a dentist will be felt long after the decision is made. Never select a dentist in the same manner you would a restaurant for a casual evening.

There's nothing casual about dentistry.

It's my experience that many people start their search for a dentist online. Google is often the place they start. However, if you type, 'Dentists Southwestern Ohio' you will be returned 987,000 results. Narrow that search to 'General Dentists Fairfield Ohio' and the resulting search presents you with 479,000 results (numbers reflected as of the writing of this book)·

The point is, if you start your search online you will have more information put in front of you than you will know what to do with. The bigger problem is which of it do you believe and more importantly, which applies to you.

Something you should know about the Internet is that it's a 'pay to play' environment. The biggest practices, with the most money, get the top rankings online. Truth be told, all that information is important, but good luck trying to find what's relevant to your specific needs, especially if you have a dental emergency and you need out of pain immediately.

When searching online for information about dentists you can become a victim of information overload. I experience it all the time when I start researching something I'm interested in. You can be left feeling overwhelmed, and having to 'figure it out', on your own.

Nothing Beats Experience AND Information Is NO Substitute For It.

What kind of experience are you looking for then? You want a professional who specializes in personal care. That may go without saying, but remember, you can easily be persuaded by fancy websites and convincing sales copy. You should always listen to your instinct. The old adage of, "If it's too good to be true then it probably is" holds true. Never doubt your first impressions.

You want a dentist who has the experience in the dental care you want and need. If you need only checkups and cleanings, who's the best? If you need more extensive treatment, who's the best and what do patients say about them. Not just from superficial testimonials and random online reviews, what are patients really saying about the care they receive.

Value and experience is something you'll recognize when you talk to the people in the practice and when you speak to the dentist. Doing the research online is okay, it's a great place to start, but you really want to talk with the people in the practice and hear from the patients who've been patients for years... and why. Just as you know when you're in love, you'll know a great practice when you know it!

When you go online and search for practices like mine you will find there are over 25 general dentists within a 5 mile radius of my practice. That's a lot less of a search result than the 479,000 you will get from Google, but the same challenge holds true. Often you will see my listings atop those searches. That's intentional. As I shared in the first chapter, I entered dentistry to help people. More specifically I want to help people save their teeth.

Regardless of which dentist you find topping the Google search, the real question you need to answer for yourself is, "Which dentist is right for you?" I would again respond with 'trust your gut'. It will require you doing some due diligence. That should include calling the practices and talking with the person who answers the phone. How are you treated?

Are you asked name, rank and serial number kind of questions or are you asked questions that are important to understanding why you're calling, for what and how they can best help you.

Do they ask you to set an appointment? A dental practice who really has your best interest in mind won't let you go without setting an appointment, at least a meet and greet with the doctor. That may sound self-serving and potentially focused on their wanting to pitch dental treatments but it's not, at the right practice. Yes, it is sometimes necessary to present you with treatment options if I find there's the need for them, but it really isn't about the money, it's more about your care and well being. Here's something you should know about most dentists, they're terrible sales people. It's not in our nature to 'sell' dentistry. It is in our nature to present dentistry and a great dentist will not present care that's not necessary. There should always be options presented with the treatment, unless your condition requires immediate attention and treatment. Even in these cases, there often are options on how to proceed. Even with the investment for treatments...there always should be options presented to you. If the doctor isn't able to give you options, then you might consider seeking a second opinion or a new dentist.

I will always be interested in meeting you and discussing your dental needs, but understand (as I do) I know I'm not the right doctor for every patient. The decision is ultimately yours and I will conclude this chapter restating that you must always trust your instinct when it comes to your health and the quality of care you receive. The final decision always rests with you. If you're not sure, ask questions and seek out people you trust.

A patient's perspective: "I haven't been to a dentist in like 20, 25 years..." - Teresa Beatty."

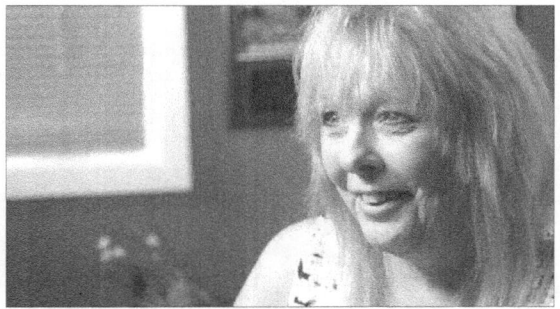

"I hadn't been to a dentist in like 20, 25 years, since I was a kid. He caters to chickens, and that's what I am. I had a really bad tooth and had tried everything, and it just ... I had to go. My whole everything just hurt. He took it out and from then on he did partial plate front dentures, and he pulled four teeth and did the plate in the same day and didn't have a problem. He just talks to you and checks every few minutes. "You all right? You all right? You all right?" Don't be afraid of him; he'll take care of that. He's a very personable person. He's good to talk to, easy, tells you everything up front, and good prices, and they help you."

I am accepting new patients. You can schedule an appointment by calling (513) 829-9700 or visiting www.DrDine.com to request an appointment online.

Dr. Andrew Dine

Chapter 8 - Brushing & Flossing

"Directions are instructions given to explain how. Direction is a vision offered to explain why." Simon Sinek

---

This is the chapter that you probably expected to be in a book from a dentist, but, it's not what you'd expect (completely), I promise.

Brushing and flossing are the curse of both dentists and patients. If you've heard it once from a dentists you've heard it a thousand times... "You should brush and floss more."

Well I both agree and disagree with that. I do believe you should brush more, but also brush better. Flossing is important, but when your mouth is healthy.

You brush to remove the particles and gunk from your teeth, and to apply the toothpaste. As you'll come to understand here, cavities are not caused by not brushing, they're caused by other factors going on in your mouth. To use an auto analogy again, here in Ohio we have cold weather in the winter. We also have snow and the cities and counties use rock salt on the roads to melt the snow. When we drive on roads that have been covered with rock salt our cars kick that salt up onto the car. We can drive the car through a car wash and it'll wash the salt from the exterior, but not from inside the door jams and hidden places the salt lies. The water and soap from the car wash can get into the same recesses where the salt lies, but in many cases the salt doesn't get washed out. The water and soap only add to the destructive nature of the salt. The result is our cars rust. Brushing your teeth does the same thing. So brushing your teeth properly won't prevent cavities or cure gum disease, only a dentist can do that.

As for flossing, you've probably heard that it can help prevent gum disease. Flossing is good to do if you have a healthy mouth already, or you have something caught between your teeth and you need to remove it. Back to the car wash analogy again. If rust has already developed along the bottom of the car door, no matter how much washing and cleaning you do it won't make the rust disappear. When you have gum disease, no amount of flossing will make it go away. Gum disease is an infection and a piece of string will not make it go away. The dentist and gum treatments can make it go away.

I recently had a patient come in with pain in her gums. After an exam I found she had a hunk of walnut shell lodge between her teeth. Many patients experience this. What typically happens is they get floss and try to remove the 'something' and what can end up happening is it gets pushed down further and further. This was the situation with my patient. In her case, flossing made her situation worse and more painful. Also, removing the particles doesn't always make your gums better either. If an infection has already set into the gums then, again, flossing won't cure the situation. Flossing is good to do if you have a healthy mouth already.

I wanted to make the difference between what you may have been led to think about brushing and flossing and what is their real purpose. A lot of advertising would have you believe the brushing and flossing is the solution to creating a healthy mouth, when in fact it's their use that allows you to maintain a healthy mouth. Once you have cavities and/or gum disease, it's the dentist that helps you eliminate it.

A dentist will tell you that you need to brush and floss more because it's the easy way out. Telling you that puts the responsibility of a healthy mouth on you. As you've already read several times, my goal is to help you have a healthy mouth. A healthy mouth is a shared responsibility between you and the dentist. The dentist gets your mouth healthy and then you maintain it with brushing and flossing.

If you have problems with your teeth and/or gums brushing and flossing more won't fix the problems. You have to get to a dentist.

Now for a brief explanation as to why you get cavities. The cause of most all problems that happen in your mouth are caused by having too much acid in your mouth. This has to do with how well balanced the acidity and alkalinity is in your mouth.

That's a battle taking place in your mouth. The foods and drinks you consume change the environment in your mouth. Your saliva works to balance the pH levels.

Not to get into a detailed lesson in chemistry, the simplest explanation is that too much acid creates an environment that promotes bad bacteria, which eats away at your teeth. A balanced or alkaline environment creates good bacteria that promotes and helps maintain a healthy mouth.

To bring things full circle from where I started this chapter, dentists tell you that you need to brush and floss more. To have a healthy mouth you first must get a healthy mouth, then brush and floss regularly. The foods and drinks you put away are delicious to devour but they are what has the most damaging effect on creating an unhealthy situation in your mouth. When you don't have the opportunity to brush after a meal, you should drink plenty of water.

Brushing and flossing are important, but they are not the 'end all - be all' cure to your dental problems. It starts with getting and maintaining a healthy mouth. For most people that means getting to the dentist, seeing your dentist at least twice a year for checkups and cleanings and then brushing and flossing more. It doesn't start with brushing and flossing more as most dentists would have you believe.

In the next chapter I'll share more details about the healthy and unhealthy mouth.

A patient's perspective: *"Checked to make sure I was all right."* - **Raymond Schmitz**

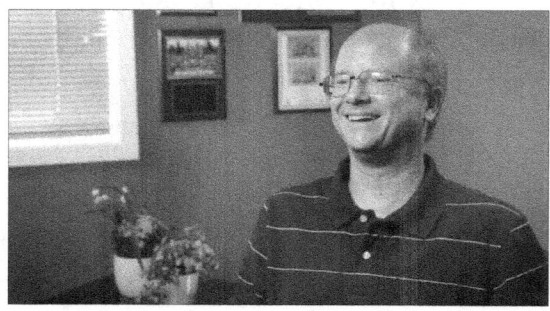

" He's a family dentist, is what I like to consider it. He does, he really cares about the individual patient, always follows up. I had a filling filled once, and he followed up a couple days later. Checked to make sure I was all right. He seems like he really cares about his patients. He really does. Wasn't painful at all. He numbs it, numbs ya. Takes care of it right then and there. It was very quick; quick turnaround to get all that done. Relatively simple office, like I said, it's not this big huge elaborate operation that's going to end up ... they throw a lot of extra cost on you when you have those big fancy places. Those things aren't free. I've always been happy with Dr. Dine. I think he does really try to keep the cost down. That matters a lot, and it's not like he's sacrificing any service for it either. In fact, I think the service is better. I like how Dr. Dine's office, they keep it a relatively small operation. It's much more personable. It's not like a big elaborate operation where you don't know what dentist you're going to see when you come in. He's the one that actually is in there working on my mouth the whole time. I appreciate that."

I am accepting new patients. You can schedule an appointment by calling (513) 829-9700 or visiting www.DrDine.com to request an appointment online.

Dr. Andrew Dine

Chapter 9 The Miracle Dental Solution

> ***"There are only two ways to live your life. One is as though nothing is a miracle. The other is as though everything is a miracle."*** Albert Einstein

---

This chapter will be an extension of the previous, though here I'm going to share what I believe is the solution to many of the dental problems you could get (or have). It's not the end all be all cure, but it's a good start for most patients. I say this from experience. I use the system I'll share and I've recommended it to many of my patients and they have success with it. My measure of their success with it is in the results I see at their biannual dental checkups.

You can only have Healthy Teeth and Gums if you understand what causes Cavities and Gum Disease. In Chapter 9 I provided you the foundational information about acidity and alkalinity in your mouth. The next thing you need to know is that Cavities and Gum Disease are diseases caused by a bacterial infection. This fact is different than the popular, but false myths concerning Cavities and Gum Disease. Basing your oral care on these myths will lead to an unhealthy mouth. Some of the biggest myths about your teeth are:

- sugar causes Cavities
- getting older causes tooth loss
- you just need to brush and floss more

I think I've already beat the message that Cavities and Gum Disease will not go away or be eliminated if you stop eating sweets and just brush and floss more. To get rid of a bacterial infection you need to eliminate the bacteria that cause the infection and disease.

There are 3 threats that are destroying your teeth and gums:

1. **Acid Mouth**
2. **Dry Mouth**
3. **Improper Home Care**

You can only eliminate these threats by knowing:

1. **Why you have Cavities and Gum Disease?**
2. **What you can do about your Cavities and Gum Disease?**
3. **How you can stop from getting Cavities and Gum Disease?**

Diseases like Cavities and Gum Disease have little or no initial symptoms. The usual sign of gum disease is when your gums bleed when you brush your teeth, but the symptoms can be present long before you see blood on your toothbrush. The only way you know if you have a cavity is if your dentist tells you or you have a hole in your tooth. Only the dentist can tell you for sure. If you ignore the obvious symptom or the advice of your dentist the consequences can be serious and lead to extensive, expensive dental treatment, or the loss of teeth.

What are the consequences of untreated Cavities and Gum Disease?

The consequences are unpleasant, uncomfortable, dangerous and painful. They include pain, infection, swelling, loss of teeth, Root Canals, Dentures, the inability to eat, missed work, sleepless nights, and connections with other serious health problems like cancer, heart disease, stroke, diabetes, lung disease, kidney disease, Alzheimer's disease and low birth weight babies. This is especially important if you're a young women looking to start a family.

What is Acid Mouth?

Acid Mouth is caused by consuming drinks and foods with an acid pH (below a pH of 7 which is water). This includes soda pop (regular and diet), fruit juices, tea and coffee, sports drinks, energy drinks, sour candies and sugar-free breath mints. Acid Mouth will also be caused by Acid Reflux disease. The bacteria that causes tooth decay needs an acidic environment to live. If you have 'Acid Mouth' you are at a high risk for Cavities. You will also have more plaque, which puts you at risk for Gum Disease. One of the great misconceptions is that once the Cavities are fixed, or you get your teeth cleaned, that is all you need to get rid of the problem. Not so! You've only eliminated the result of the underlying problem. Tooth Decay and Gum Disease are diseases and just getting your Cavities fixed, or getting your teeth cleaned, does not get rid of the disease that caused them.

What is Dry Mouth?

A Dry Mouth, which is caused with age, medications (prescription and nonprescription drugs), hormonal changes, sinus problems, allergies, sleep apnea and mouth breathing, Diabetes, Sjogren's Syndrome, radiation treatments, smoking and alcohol. These all will put you at risk for Tooth Decay and Gum Disease. You need saliva to neutralize the acid in your mouth, otherwise your teeth end up bathing in acid 24/7. At night you naturally have less saliva production. Have you ever woken up with a dry mouth? The greatest damage is done at night. With a Dry Mouth food sticks to your teeth and is hard to remove, especially along the gum line. As you sleep that nasty bacteria has the chance to eat away at your teeth and gums in a environment helpful to speeding along cavities and gum decease.

Your Home Care

Your home care is very important in the fight against Acid Mouth, Dry Mouth, Tooth Decay and Gum Disease. Unless you are utilizing the right products in the correct manner, and understand what effect your diet is having in your mouth you will lose the battle. The best home care system I have found was created by Dr. Ellie Phillips. I use this system twice a day.

It is a method of cleaning your teeth and gums in such a way that rebalances the ph level in your mouth. The harmful bacteria are eliminated and healthy bacteria are promoted.

Home care is only one part of the equation. In addition to the proper home care, you need to get your Cavities and Gum Disease treated, change your diet and start using Xylitol mints and gum to help prevent Cavities, Dry Mouth, Acid Mouth and Gum Disease. The result are cleaner, healthier teeth and gums... for a lifetime!

There is Hope - The Dine Method

I'm not a dietitian or therapist, I'm a dentist. I can only prescribe what will help you dentally. I'm going to share with you my exclusive system for helping patients. Notice I didn't say treating them. Treatment takes place when you're in my office, which often is only twice a year for most patients. That's a small percentage of time I get to see, diagnose and treat you. The majority of care takes place on your own, away from the office.

The Dine Method is a two-step system. The first part is your home care (or self care). This you do on your own. It can be at home, at work or when you're on vacation.

The home care portion of my method is based on Dr. Ellie's Complete Mouth Care System. Each step in the system has a specific purpose. The products work in harmony with one another in order to produce quick results.

You use the system twice a day (as I do). The system can be used by patients when they've gained their adult, permanent teeth. Children can use this system as young as 6-7 years old, though I recommend they be supervised until they can safely rinse and spit.

The System **

Step One - Clean

It is important to brush teeth in a neutral pH or alkaline mouth because teeth are soft in an acidic mouth and more likely to be damaged by abrasive toothpaste. Using a pH balancing rinse like CloSYS™ before brushing neutralizes teeth and loosens food particles so brushing is more effective. Do not use any flavoring in this rinse, as it will reduce the beneficial effects.

After rinsing with CloSYS™ for a minute, brush your teeth using a well-designed soft toothbrush. Be sure to brush your gums, and don't forget your six front teeth at gum level – upper and lower. Many people turn their wrists as they brush and miss these front teeth. Also take care to brush the gum on the inside of back molars along the side of your tongue.

For best results, use a soft bristle toothbrush with a head that fits your mouth and basic sodium fluoride toothpaste like Crest® Cavity Protection Toothpaste. Do not use a paste with <u>whitening agents, tartar control additives, stannous fluoride, sodium monofluorophosphate, or triclosan</u>. It is vital to disinfect your toothbrush after brushing by dipping it in Listerine® Antiseptic. If bacteria are irritating your gums, brushing may make them bleed. This is part of the healing process. If this happens; just gently brush the area that bleeds.

Step Two - Disinfect

Immediately after brushing, rinse your mouth with Listerine®, an antibacterial rinse effective against immature plaque bacteria. Use a Listerine® that carries an ADA shield of acceptance. Do not use Listerine® that advertises plaque or tartar control, or whitening, which do not carry the ADA shield of acceptance. If the rinse seems too strong– **you can dilute with water until you're used to it.**

Step Three - Protect

The final rinse is fluoride, which helps re-mineralize and strengthen teeth. We recommend ACT ® Anticavity Fluoride mouthwash. Avoid ACT ® Restore since it contains alcohol and has a different fluoride concentration. Fluoride should be kept on teeth as long as possible so it's best to rinse immediately before bed and after eating in the morning.

All Day – Get the Power of Xylitol

Xylitol is a delicious weapon in the fight against dental disease. It looks and tastes like sugar but has 40% fewer calories. When xylitol dissolves in your mouth, it makes a sweet sugary solution that is alkaline, the opposite of damaging acidic. Studies show that eating two teaspoons of xylitol each day (6-10 grams) for 5 weeks will remove harmful germs from plaque on your teeth and in 6 months 95% of these germs will be removed from your mouth.

100% xylitol mints or gum after meals, drinks and snacks is an important part of the preventative steps you can take in combating cavities and gum disease.

All of these products can be purchased in retail stores, with the exception of the Xylitol. What is missing when you purchase the items individually is my professional advice and instruction. I do have starter kits available in the office. Patients receive a kit with their gum treatments in my office. If your gums are bleeding then you should consider scheduling a gum examination. If you're in my area (the Greater Cincinnati, Ohio area) you can call my office at (513) 829-9700 to schedule an appointment.

Now, for the second step in the Dine Method, regular checkups. I'm sure that comes as no surprise. You must see a dentist at least every 6 months. Great dental care is a relationship between you and your dentist. If you don't have a dentist or aren't seeing one regularly, I'd be happy to meet you and discuss how I can help you eliminate the 3 threats that are destroying your teeth and gums.

Why should you make an appointment to meet me?

- You have pain or discomfort
- You're embarrassed to smile
- You're scared of the dentist
- You can't eat the food you love
- You want realistic solutions for your mouth
- You want a beautiful smile quickly, that won't break the bank
- You finally want someone who will care and listen
- You've had negative dental experiences in the past and you don't want to repeat them

Call my office at (513) 829-9700 to schedule a worry-free, no guilt appointment

** Borrowed directly from Dr Ellie's material

A patient's perspective: *"He doesn't talk down to you."* Angie Fisher

"This is one of the few practices where I have kept coming back. I have this, I know it's unconditional, fear of the dentist. I've jumped around to several different dentists, and this is the one where I've kept coming back, and I'm actually to the point now where I don't have to have somebody come with me. Even cleanings were a stress point for me, and they're not anymore, which is amazing.

He doesn't talk down to you. I've had experiences where a lot of dentists get frustrated easy when you maybe have a low pain tolerance, and he doesn't do that. He's very considerate, he's always asking, "Hey, is everything okay? Let me know if you feel anything," and a lot of dentists don't do that these days. He always tells me to let him know if I feel anything, and I don't feel like I'm frustrating him when I say, "Oh, wait, I feel that."

I feel like I'm taking better care of myself, where before I was so ashamed, and I had to get a different dentist for every different thing that I had going on that it didn't give me that accomplishment feeling. To where now I'm like, "Oh yeah, I got that down. Okay, this is next," and it just makes you want to come back. It makes you feel like you're actually accomplishing something with your health because your teeth have a lot to do with the overall health of your body.

If you've ever had that fear, ashamed of being afraid, don't be. They're going to welcome you with open arms and help you through it. Not just say, "Okay, let's get her in and get her out," but they actually help you with that fear, which is really good."

I am accepting new patients. You can schedule an appointment by calling (513) 829-9700 or visiting www.DrDine.com to request an appointment online.

Dr. Andrew Dine

Chapter 10 - The Dreaded Cost of Dentistry - It's really not as bad as you think

"Is money the most important thing in life?" Mother Theresa

In everyday language and conversation with others, cost, price and value are often used interchangeably. For the purpose of discussion here I want to define them.

Value:

Value is the usefulness or desirability of product or service. How much do you love it, or what it is worth to you? Value is not a number, but often you can compare the values of two things, especially if they appear to be similar to one another. For example, in dentistry you can drive down the street and see one dental practice sign after another. From the curb every dentist is the same because from your perspective at that point (driving by) they're all dentists, they all do the same thing...clean and take care of teeth. Intuitively you see their values as being fundamental. It's not until you do further investigation that you find that dentists are not all the same. Each has their own unique benefits, but the real difference between them really lies more with you than the dentist. Your individual preferences about how the dentists has decorated his or her office, how you're treated by the dentist and his or her staff. What's their personality like. Are you treated like a number on a dental chart or welcomed into the practice as one of the family?

This value has little to do with how much a dental procedures costs. You could have the cheapest dentist in town and be treated like an insignificant member of society, or you could invest a little extra and be treated with respect and dignity. The choice is yours, and your pocketbook is not the best measuring tool for this criteria. (I would refer you back to Chapter 2)

It's impossible to ever put a price on value. Value is relative. Your value of something will be entirely different than that of a friend or family member.

Cost or Price

I believe cost and price are interchangeable. This has to do with the amount of money required to purchase something (a good or a service). In today's society of instant information cost is often a negative thing because one can get a price or cost of something almost instantly. With the commoditization of many things we're conditioned to always think we can get something cheaper elsewhere. In a lot of national dentistry advertising the public is led to believe they can shop for dentistry as any other other commodity like facial tissue. However, when you have a severe sinus cold and your nose is running and you're having to blow your nose continually, you'll pay the extra price for the facial tissue made with Aloe Vera because it makes a difference on your comfort than wiping with that toilet paper grade tissue. There's the difference between value and price.

Hygiene for example is a service you can get in most dental practices. However, the quality of your cleaning, the relationship with the hygienist and whether you go home feeling like he or she cleaned your teeth with a jack hammer and chisel or by the gentle caress of caring hands skilled with the tools. The difference between price and value.

Now for the reality, dentistry isn't cheap and it shouldn't be. We're talking about your health, not just your teeth. If your child had a brain injury you wouldn't seek out the cheapest brain surgeon. If your mother had a heart condition you wouldn't want the cheapest heart surgeon. "But Dr. Dine, dentistry isn't brain or heart surgery." Not entirely, but the quality of your dental health has a direct impact on every other part of your body. The Chinese have a saying "Disease enters through the mouth." Yet it appears that many doctors do not like this concept.

So what about dental insurance?

As a dentist I'm trained to provide excellent care and service and to make people's mouths healthy. Yet there is a lot that gets in the way of that financially for some people. I believe there is a general belief that dental insurance should be like medical insurance, but it's not.

Unfortunately insurance providers do not give dental care the same weight they give medical care. However most medical insurance is designed to cover what adjusters call 'catastrophic incidents'. That would be heart attacks, strokes, cancer, etc. Life altering conditions. Granted, I realize that's a broad statement. In fact, most medical insurance is applied to much more routine situations like health checkups and the such. Comparing medical insurance to dental insurance is like comparing apples to watermelons. Medical insures treatment and care for a much broader spectrum of care. Medical insurance in general is for treating all other parts of the body (physically and sometimes mentally) except for the mouth. It's for virtually everything head to toe. In short, it's all encompassing. Medical and dental insurance cannot be compared equally. With nearly all medical and dental insurances you will have deductibles and out of pocket expenses. With dental insurance there is a maximum benefit each year. Every plan is different. You should know the benefits available to you under your plan.

There is a difference between insurance costs and deductible costs. Insurance premiums is how much it costs to have insurance and deductibles and co-pays are how much it costs to use the insurance. According to national research many consumers face deductibles of $3000 or more. Under the Affordable Care Act, deductibles in Ohio have risen[3] from $375 to $583 on top of those already steep deductible rates. With an ever aging population those cost will continue to increase. To make matters worse, rates and deductibles are expected to continue to skyrocket further during 2017 and 2018 under the Affordable Care Act.

Let's compare two medical procedures to see really how much things cost. I'll compare a carpal tunnel relief surgery versus a root canal. I chose these two to compare because A) they're both predominately pain-relief procedures; B) they're comparatively the same with regard to the treatment time for the patient, and C) carpal tunnel and root canal procedures are generally covered under insurance. I'm trying to provide an apples to apples comparison between a medical and dental treatment, not a cost-to-cost comparison.

Carpal Tunnel Relief Surgery

A recent study published in the Proceedings of the National Academy of Sciences found that only 14% of Americans understood their own insurance policy. According to the American Insurance Institute the national average out-of-pocket cost on carpal tunnel surgery is $4,426, and that's if you are insured and your insurance covers the treatment. Actual cost for the treatment can range from $3,011 to $7,202 per hand. Aftercare (if needed) can double those figures. To be completely transparent, that $4,426 national average breaks down as $1,182 for the surgery and $3,244 for post operative expenses[4].

Root Canal Procedure

The cost of a root canal can vary depending on the dentist. Unlike carpal tunnel, teeth vary based on the number of roots they have and this dictates the cost of a procedure. For a canine or incisor the range for treatment is $400 to $1,000. A multi-rooted tooth, such as molars and premolars can cost $500 to $2,000 per tooth[6]. So the average out-of-pocket costs for patients with insurance, for a root canal is $700 to $1,180 and no post operative expenses.

The point being, both procedures covered by insurance, medical and dental, and both having real out-of-pocket expenses for the patient.

According to an article in the New York Times (December 1, 2016) more than 500,000 people in the US undergo carpal tunnel surgery[6]. According to the American Association of Endodontists on average Endodontists perform 41,000 root canals a day[7] and nearly 15 million per year. Some general dentists are trained to perform root canals. I perform root canals, but I provided information from the American Association of Endodontists because information specific to root canal procedures performed is much more accurate.

(Endodontists are specialists who treat specific problems with the tissues inside the tooth, which includes the roots.)

When you compare apples to apples, medical and dental insurances are similar in the respect of what a patient ultimately pays out-of-pocket. The difference is more in mindset than reality. Most people don't feel the out-of-pocket pain when they go to the physician because most visits are routine and the only out-of-pockets are their co-pays, which can be as low as $15 depending on one's plan. Despite daily reports in the media about a person diagnosed with some terrible ailment most people's physician visits are pretty benign. In most cases people are taking care of their bodies. On the other hand, when one visits the dentist we seem to be the bearer of bad news more frequently. Why? Refer back to Chapters 8 & 9. People take less care of their teeth and the results can be expected. Sir Isaac Newton's third law was, "For every action there is an equal and opposite reaction".

So what does all this mean? Dental care and treatment is not as expensive as one might have you believe. If you recall earlier in the chapter I shared that only 14% of Americans understood their insurance policies? Truth be told, in my experience most people don't fully maximize the dental insurance they do have. Your dental office should be helping you maximize your plan's benefits so that you receive all the treatment you're paying for. Let me say that a different way. You should be maximizing your benefits so you get all the treatment you're entitled to. If you're not taking full advantage of the dental insurance benefits available to you then you're wasting money. You're paying money to an insurance company and not getting the service you've paid for, because you're not using it.

Additionally, when a patient has exceeded their benefits and treatment exceeds the money their plan allows, most dental practices offer other financing options. In some cases, they make arrangements internally with patients. Despite what some may think of dentists, we still think and operate like those dentists who used to make house calls to their patients; when they had the patient's best interest in mind.

There are any number of ways to make your dental care and treatment affordable. I do it in my office. If you're at a practice that doesn't have your best interest in mind, both medically and financially then a change of practice may be in order.

When it comes to dentistry, you either have a price or value attitude. There are different dental practices for each type of patient. My patients tend to have a value attitude and we work the rest out.

Resources:
[3] http://www.nationalreview.com/article/433940/obamacare-deductibles-are-skyrocketing-affordable-care-act-health-insurance-anything
[4] http://www.carpalrx.com/surgery-and-insurance
[5] http://budgeting.thenest.com/average-cost-root-canal-good-insurance-28427.html
[6] http://www.nytimes.com/health/guides/disease/carpal-tunnel-syndrome/surgery.html
[7] http://www.aae.org/about-aae/news-room/endodontic-facts.aspx

---

A patient's perspective: "That's one thing that's really important." Ginger Bryd

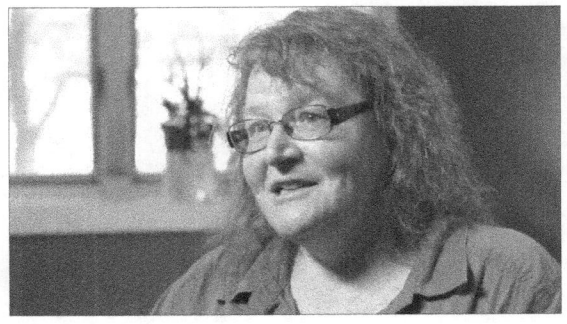

"Dr. Dine is personable. He basically is always friendly, he greets you, he shakes your hand, he thanks you for coming. He even follows up, like after a procedure, he will call you. He'll say, how did everything go, are you feeling okay, are you in pain – he'll call you the next day to make sure you are okay, which is something totally different.

They very seldom ever have you waiting more than just a few minutes at the most. That's one thing that is really important.

They're always friendly, they always give you a reminder call when it's time for your appointment. I've always gotten along really well with them, they're always very nice.

He would always say, are you doing okay, hold up your hand if you're in pain or if you need to rinse or whatever, so yes, he was very conscientious about that.

Sometimes I notice that he has different procedures that he uses and stuff so I'm sure he goes back and has some re-training and learns some new things as he goes along too. He's trying to keep up to date, which is a good thing.

They're very professional. They treat you well; I've never had any issues at all, they've always been really good to me."

I am accepting new patients. You can schedule an appointment by calling (513) 829-9700 or visiting www.DrDine.com to request an appointment online.

Chapter 11 - Treating Patients

"Do what you can, with what you have, where you are." Theodore Roosevelt

This chapter is the chapter you'd expect to be in this book. You'll notice however I've saved it for near the end. I did so intentionally because as you've no doubt discovered from the previous chapters, I'm not your ordinary dentist. My focus has always been on the patient.

I am however, regardless of my approach to the science, still a general dentist. I would not be doing myself, or you as my patient, a service if you weren't aware of what treatments you can and should expect from your dentist. As you investigate dental practices (and general dentists), what they offer can vary with regard to the services. At some practices the dentist will perform most of the services within the practice. He or she will perform the procedures themselves or bring a specialist in, based on the frequency of need for specialized services, like root canals. Other dentists will refer specialized services out. They do so either because they are not trained in or proficient at certain specialized treatments.

You should decide in advance how you want your dentist to provide the services you will need, or potentially need in the future. Here's a a general idea of the services I provide patients in my practice.

Dental Cleanings and Exams:

The most important thing you can do for the health and well-being of your smile is get routine dental cleanings and dental exams.

Why Dental Cleanings and Dental Exams Are Important

There are two major reasons that professional dental cleanings and dental exams at our office are important for the health of your smile.

- *Prevention* – Catching issues early on gives us the best chance to treat them successfully. By identifying potential problems before they become serious, we can effectively treat them.
- *Hygiene* – Whether you brush your teeth for 10 minutes or 10 hours, you will still miss areas of your teeth. Professional dental cleanings and dental exams will help us find those areas and remove the plaque and tartar buildup.

Your First Dental Visit

On your first visit we'll get the chance to meet each other and discuss what you want to accomplish with your dental care.

On your hygiene visit I will give your teeth a thorough cleaning and look for any signs of gum disease, oral cancer, tooth decay, and more. I also will take digital X-rays. Though I use a lot of state-of-the-art technology, I don't ignore the tried and true methods for improving the health of your teeth.

Should I find something, I will work with you to develop a treatment plan and get your smile back to a healthy mouth, based on your needs and budget.

I Make Your First Visit Free from Dental Anxiety

Some people have concerns about visiting the dentist. They might worry about comfort, costs, or similar problems. At our office, we understand that you might have had bad experiences in the past. That's why we are dedicated to doing what we can to put you at ease. We offer pain-free local anesthesia with Dental Vibe, effortless cleaning with ultrasonic, and nitrous oxide (laughing gas) when appropriate.

Cosmetic Dentistry:

Here are some of the fast and effective cosmetic dentistry services we offer you.
- *Dental veneers*
- *Teeth whitening*
- *Invisalign*

The Benefits of Invisalign Adult Orthodontics

- *Discreet Appearance* – No worrying about what metal brackets look like on your teeth, because with Invisalign braces, there are no visible signs of your straightening efforts. Your clear plastic aligners are nearly invisible to other people, allowing you to straighten your smile discreetly.
- *Convenience* – Your Invisalign orthodontic aligners are removable, so there's no changing your diet or your oral hygiene routine. You can eat what you want, when you want. You can also brush and floss your teeth the same way you always have.
- *Comfort* – The smooth plastic will not injure the inside of your mouth, and there are no sharp edges to eat or talk around. You will barely even know your invisible braces are there. Trust your smile to Invisalign from Dr. Dine. Call our office for your orthodontic consultation now.

What Is Invisalign Preview?

Invisalign preview lets us show you what your smile is going to look like at the end of your treatment. At your Invisalign consultation, we'll start by taking photos of your smile and dental impressions to record the exact positions of your teeth. We send this information to Invisalign. Invisalign sends back a computer-generated simulation that will show you how your teeth will move during your treatment and a sneak preview of your new smile! At our office, there's no guesswork with your orthodontic treatment.

What You Need to Know About the Invisalign Process

There are a few important things to know about your Invisalign treatment:
- You wear your aligner trays at least 20 hours per day for best smile results
- You move to the next aligner set in your series every two weeks
- You get your new smile in as little as 12 months!

The Benefits of Cosmetic Dentistry

- *Appearance* – With teeth whitening, dental veneers, and tooth bonding, we can make your teeth look better and help you feel good about the appearance of your smile.
- *Confidence* – The boost to your self-confidence is remarkable when you finally get the attractive smile you have always wanted.
- *Oral Health* – In addition to your appearance, cosmetic dentistry services like Invisalign and dental veneers can improve your oral health. Straight teeth are easier to clean, and dental veneers will protect cracked teeth from cracking any further.

Dental Crowns and Bridges:

A damaged or missing tooth can cause you a lot of pain, but dental crowns and bridges from Dr. Dine can repair your smile and relieve your pain. Trust a dentist who has spent 40 years helping patients just like you get back to eating and smiling comfortably again. I use Zirconia to give you some of the strongest, most natural-looking crowns and bridges possible.

When Would You Need a Dental Crown?

Dental crowns are an amazingly versatile tool for repairing your damaged tooth. Dental crowns restore the look and function of your teeth. Here is when you may need their help.

- *Cracked Teeth* – Moderate to severe cracks need a dental crown to keep them from breaking apart fully.
- *Broken Teeth* – To save you from needing an extraction, Dr. Dine may use a dental crown to protect your broken tooth.
- *Root Canal Treatment* – Dental crowns are often used to restore your tooth after a root canal.
- *Severe Tooth Decay* – When your tooth decay does not leave enough of your natural tooth to support a filling, dental crowns are a great option.

When you lose a tooth, you need to find something to fill that void in your smile. Dental bridges are able to complete your smile. By using dental crowns to anchor a replacement tooth into your smile, I will repair your appearance and restore your mouth to full function. Enjoy your food with ease again!

Dental Implants:

If you are missing teeth or are going to have damaged teeth

removed, Dr. Dine has a tooth replacement solution for you. Dental implants are able to fully replace your natural tooth and give you superior stability, longevity, and function when compared to other options.

What Is a Dental Implant?

I often recommend dental implants to replace your natural tooth roots. A dental implant is gently inserted into the area left empty from your natural tooth. It bonds with your jawbone to give you a stable foundation for your new tooth.

After having your implant placed by one of our trusted oral surgeon partners, Dr. Dine will create and attach a dental crown to complete your smile and restore your appearance.

Benefits of Dental Implants from Dr. Dine

- *Stability* – The titanium of the dental implant is able to fully bond with the bone in your jaw. This process is called osseointegration and is critical to how effective dental implants are for our patients.
- *Longevity* – Today's dental implants can conceivably last you a lifetime with proper care and regular visits to our office.
- *Appearance* – Your smile will look as good or even better than it did before you lost your natural tooth. The solid Zirconia dental crown that Dr. Dine places will look and feel just like your real tooth did. Zirconia is an amazingly strong material that reflects light in the same way as your real teeth. An implant will look and act just like your real tooth, so you can be confident in your smile again.

Dentures:

Dentures are a great way to replace several missing teeth with a single solution. With options that range from full dentures to partial dentures and even implant-supported dentures

With a number of different options and four decades of experience, we are equipped to handle whatever your dental needs are.

Types of Dentures

- *Partial Dentures* – When you only need a few teeth replaced, partial dentures from Dr. Dine are a solution that will work well for you and your smile.
- *Full Dentures* – For patients who need a full arch of teeth replaced, full dentures are a wonderful option. They are less expensive and less invasive than dental implants.
- *Implant-Supported Dentures* – Stabilize your dentures with the help of dental implants. Instead of relying only on suction and denture adhesives, these dentures use a bar attachment to connect to implants surgically placed in your jawbone. The stability these dentures provide mean you can eat what you want, speak to whomever you want, and smile freely knowing your dentures are going to stay right where they are supposed to. Ask our Fairfield, OH dentist if implant-supported dentures will work well for you.

Non Surgical Gum Disease Treatment:

What Is Gum Disease?

Periodontal disease, or gum disease, is an infection within your gum tissue caused by bacteria buildup. Eventually, it can

damage your bone if left untreated. Here are signs of gum disease.
- *Bleeding Gums*
- *Red, Inflamed Gum Tissue*
- *Gum pockets around your teeth*
- The consequences of gum disease include:
- *Gum Recession*
- *Loose and Shifting Teeth*
- *Tooth Loss*

Effective Gum Disease Treatments from Dr. Andrew Dine, DDS

Gum Treatments- Dr. Dine will perform professional gum treatments to remove the tartar, plaque and infection that is under your gums. To insure your comfort, Dr. Dine will numb the area and Nitrous Oxide is available to help you relax and feel-at-ease.

Antibiotics – As with any bacterial infection, antibiotics can help eliminate the bacteria and rid your mouth of the damaging periodontal infection.

Root Canal:

There are a lot of rumors and myths about root canal treatment. At Andrew Dine, DDS, your root canal will not hurt, and it may be the only way to save your damaged tooth from extraction. With our skills and advanced techniques like DentalVibe, you can have a painless root canal experience and keep your beautiful smile intact.

Why Would You Need a Root Canal?

A root canal is needed if an infection has reached the inner chamber of the tooth that houses the dental pulp. The dental pulp consists of blood vessels that nourish the tooth as well as nerves that trigger pain when irritated. If infection is left untreated, it will kill the dental pulp, destroy bone, and spread to surrounding areas. This will lead to you losing the tooth and requiring a bridge or dental implant to fill the gap.

How Do You Know If You Need a Root Canal?

If you experience any of the following symptoms of dental pulp infection, do not wait. Call your dentist in Fairfield, OH right away:
- Severe toothache that may disappear and return
- Pain when chewing or biting
- Prolonged sensitivity to hot and cold
- Tooth discoloration
- Persistent bad breath
- Pus-filled abscess near the aching tooth
- Loose teeth

However, you may notice no symptoms at all. That's why it's so important to have regular dental cleanings and exams, so Dr. Dine has the opportunity to catch any infection before it spreads.

What Is the Root Canal Process?

Before anything happens, I will use my painless Dental Vibe technology to completely numb the tooth and surrounding tissue so you won't feel anything. Once the area is numb, I can start your root canal treatment. It sounds worse than it actually is.

The purpose of the root canal is remove the damaged nerve

and pulp. The tooth is cleaned out, and the inside is filled with gutta-percha (a material similar to the removed pulp). Depending on the extent of the damage, I may seal your tooth with a tooth-colored filling or dental crown to repair your tooth and make it strong again.

Sedation Options for Anxious Patients:

For more than four decades, I have been helping patients have comfortable, calm trips to the dentist. Nitrous oxide dental sedation is a great way to take the edge off your nerves before your dental treatment.

The Benefits of Dental Sedation

- *Speed* – Nitrous oxide takes effect fast. It will only take a moment for you to begin feeling the effects of the sedative. With nitrous, also known as laughing gas, you will feel slightly drowsy but will still be able to participate as needed in your treatment. Nitrous also wears off quickly following your appointment, so you won't need someone to drive you home.
- *Comfort* – The euphoric sensation that accompanies nitrous oxide is what many patients need to get their dental care completed. While it doesn't numb your body, it certainly takes the edge off your senses and makes everything a lot more comfortable. We can adjust it at any time during your procedure, making it a safe way to ensure your comfort throughout your visit.

When Is Nitrous Oxide Sedation Used?

Nitrous oxide is a relatively mild sedative. This makes it very versatile for different dental treatments and for different

ages. Here are some ways we help our patients with dental sedation.
- *Routine Cleanings*
- *Deep Cleaning for Gum Disease*
- *Receiving a Dental Filling*
- *Getting Root Canal Treatment*
- *Having a Tooth Extracted*
- *Completing Multiple Treatments in One Easy Visit*

Teeth Whitening:

The color of your teeth has a dramatic impact on the appearance of your smile. That impact is a positive one. Patients are often surprised to discover how inexpensive and speedy a professionally whitened smile can be when combined with your routine dental cleaning and exam

Sinsational Smile Fast Teeth Whitening

My 'Sinsational Smile' system can give you an amazingly whiter smile in as little as 20 minutes. All it takes is three easy steps:
- *Step #1* – Vitamin E is applied to your lips to protect them during your teeth whitening treatment.
- *Step #2* – The custom trays and whitening solution are placed on your teeth. You will get to take the trays home with a special whitening pen for easy touch-ups in between teeth whitening treatments.
- *Step #3* – A special L.E.D. light is applied to your teeth. This activates and enhances the whitening effects of the whitening gel.

At the end, you will have a whiter smile (in as little as 20 minutes) and have none of the tooth or gum sensitivity other treatments produce, thanks to our professional system.

Professional Teeth Whitening vs. Over-the-Counter Teeth Whitening

You can spend anywhere from $20 to $100 for an OTC teeth whitening solution that will take a week or more to show only minimal results. Or you can spend about the same amount for a professional teeth whitening solution here and have some amazing results in 20 minutes – plus, the added benefit of do it yourself at-home touch-ups!

Teeth Removal and Extractions:

It's my last resort, but sometimes removing teeth is necessary to keep your smile healthy. I have decades of experience and the skills to make sure your smile is taken care of properly. With my DentalVibe technology and dental sedation that will make your procedure painless, I will have you on the road to a better smile in no time.

"Well, I went through cancer treatments, and we ended up taking all my teeth out. See, now I got all new teeth. I had no smile. Now, I have a smile. I started coming to him about 20 years ago, and I told him then, I didn't really think that they were worth saving, and he said, "Oh, no, we've got to save them," so we tried, but probably maybe would've succeeded until the leukemia, and then the chemo just screwed up the works. So they just were falling out on about a five week average, every, I'd lose one. I only had like 11 teeth left, anyway. So now at least I can chew stuff. Even when I had teeth, he was very good about the painkillers and stuff like that, as far as shots and ... You didn't feel anything. If you felt something, he was like, "Okay, we'll stop. We'll get that squared away." He was really aware of that.

Sometimes, I wouldn't even say anything. He goes, "You felt that, didn't you?" I go, "Yeah, yeah." "Okay, well I'll get..." you know ... Simple, painless, never felt anything." Chuck B.

Here are some Common Reasons for a Tooth Extraction

- *Severe Tooth Decay* – Tooth decay eats away at your tooth and can spread to other teeth nearby. When too much of your tooth has been damaged for a filling or dental crown, a dental extraction may be necessary. If you have a bad toothache, call us right away.
- *Broken Tooth* – A broken tooth may not be able to be saved. Dr. Dine can safely remove the tooth and give you the pain relief you need.
- *Crowded Mouth* – It's possible your mouth cannot accommodate all your teeth. To alleviate this crowding, Dr. Dine can strategically remove a tooth to create space for a more balanced smile.

Tooth Colored Fillings:

Tooth-colored fillings allow me to repair your tooth and get them back to being healthy without the unsightly traditional silver mercury fillings.

Why Would I Need a Tooth Filling?

You may need a tooth filling if you suffer from mild to moderate tooth decay (cavity). Tooth decay eats away at your tooth and won't stop unless I remove the destroyed part of your tooth. I use composite resin dental fillings to repair the destroyed part and seal your tooth from bacteria.

Benefits of Composite Resin Tooth Fillings

- *Biocompatible* – The composite resin we use for your tooth filling chemically bonds with your tooth, which will keep it strong for years.
- *Blends in with your natural smile* – Dr. Dine can shade your composite resin tooth filling to match your existing teeth exactly. This will leave your filling practically undetectable.
- *Requires less tooth removal than with metal fillings* – Dental enamel doesn't grow back, so the less we have to remove for your filling, the more healthy tooth we can preserve.
- *Less sensitivity than metal fillings*
- *Strengthens the walls of the tooth*
- *Shaped to resemble your natural tooth*

Dental Veneers:

Dental veneers are a tremendous tool when it comes to transforming the look of your teeth. I have more than 40 years of cosmetic dentistry experience and have crafted a perfect dental smile with veneers for quite a few patients. Whether suffering from cracked, chipped, or stained teeth, dental veneers can often correct your problems in just one visit.

Composite Dental Veneers Make a Huge Impact on Your Smile

A dental veneer is a thin piece of composite resin that is molded in the shape of your tooth. Here are some of the cosmetic dentistry issues we can correct with composite veneers.

- *Chipped Teeth*
- *Cracked Teeth*
- *Misshapen Teeth*

- *Stained Teeth*
- *Gaps Between Teeth*

Benefits of Composite Dental Veneers

- *Less Prep Work* – Porcelain dental veneers require the removal of a thin layer of dental enamel before they're applied. That's why I offer composite dental veneers. There is little to no tooth enamel removal required for this type of dental veneer, which leaves your tooth more naturally intact.
- *More affordable* – Composite veneers can be potentially half the cost of porcelain veneers. I think you should be able to have a great smile without breaking the bank.
- *Fast Application* – With traditional porcelain veneers, you wait weeks for them to be made before they can be applied to your teeth. With veneers, the same day you walk in for your composite dental veneer, you will walk out with your veneer. There is no waiting for your new smile here.

If you read through the whole list of services I provide you should be saying to yourself, "That's a lot", and it is. You should not be surprised to know I do all the work myself. Often patients think because I do the work myself they're waiting a long time, and you're not.

A Patient's Perspective: *"It's a very efficient, very professional office "*
Jennifer Reid

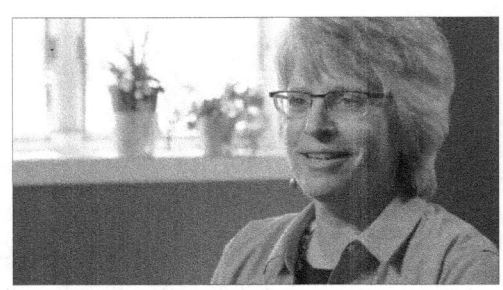

"I never have to wait. I know that might seem like maybe something that shouldn't be a top priority but I just think it's intolerable to sit in a doctor's office for thirty minutes, an hour, an hour and a half. I've gone to dentists before where I had to wait a really long time, and as a matter of fact, he kind of set a standard for me. I don't wait for any doctors anymore. If Dr. Dine can do it, then everybody else can too. My general practitioner, I don't wait for him anymore, but Dr. Dine helped me set that as a standard.

I find them to be very efficient, very professional. I think Dr. Dine continues to discover the latest technology, and the latest training, he goes to seminars and workshops, conferences, that type of thing. He's has a very pleasant personality, the staff, they're all very pleasant, very caring people. While you don't wait and his procedures don't take a lot of time, I never feel like I'm being rushed through, like sometimes I felt.

I'm going to use the word engaged to describe Dr. Dine. Because he always seems to me to be very engaging with me personally. He's very engaged with his staff. You get the sense after this many years that this isn't just a sterile, cold work environment. There is a family here of sorts, there really is.

He's really engaged in his work, and in his profession and learning more about it and wanting to be the best that he can be in his profession. He doesn't just sit back and coast the way some of us might do professionally as the years goes by. He still comes across as, maybe not the new kid on the block, but somebody who still has a lot to learn and wants to learn it and wants to be the best that he can be." Jennifer Reid

If you polled all my patients and asked what they find most refreshing here it would be that I am a no nonsense doctor. I will tell you like it is, but I also will never make you feel guilty or ashamed for the current state of your teeth. If you've not been able to care for them as you should or would like, that's okay. It's not my place to shame you into anything or make you feel ashamed for anything you haven't done. I'm not a monster, I'm a person just like you, and there are things my doctors tell me I should do too and I don't.

I am accepting new patients. You can schedule an appointment by calling (513) 829-9700 or visiting www.DrDine.com to request an appointment online.

Dr. Andrew Dine

Chapter 12 - Your Journey

"A journey of a thousand miles begins with one step." Lao Tzu (Chinese philosopher)

As trivial as Tzu's quote is, it couldn't be more true. A journey of a thousand miles or just the journey in finding the dentist that's right for you, successfully navigating that journey requires steps... the right steps. The actress Meryl Streep said: *"Start by starting."* Getting started is often the hardest part. You've already done that, by reading this book.

As I stated at the end of the opening chapter, my mission as a dentist is to get every patient to a healthy mouth. My mission as the author of this book is to offer you the tools needed to find a dentist who will get you to a healthy mouth.

If you're in the Southwestern or Greater Cincinnati, Ohio area then I would hope that both the dentist and author in me can help you. That means having you as a patient in my practice. I'd welcome the opportunity to meet you. If your thinking and mine align then I think it would be mutually beneficial that we meet.

If you're new to the area and are looking for a dentist, or, you're currently seeing a dentist and have been thinking about changing practices (for reasons I don't need to know about) or you would like to get a second opinion on a treatment plan presented to you, then I'm available to help. You simply call my office in Fairfield, Ohio at (513) 829-9700 to schedule an appointment. You also can request an appointment online at www.drdine.com. I understand how patients can feel about scheduling an appointment. The idea of seeing a dentist can be overwhelming and the idea of calling the office to schedule can be overwhelming. If you feel that way too, take comfort in knowing I've had several patients who felt the same. That's why I make the online process available. I can't help you if I don't meet you.

If you have any questions that I haven't answered in this book, you also can call my office at (513) 829-9700 and I or my assistant will be more than happy to answer all your questions. I can guarantee that you will have a completely enjoyable experience here, as a patient, as you've read from many of my patients throughout this book.

If you're not in my neck of the woods, then I hope I've accomplished my goal of giving you the tools needed to seek out a competent, caring, compassionate dentist whose first interest is your best interest as a patient, not his or her bottom line. The journey to finding the dentist who is right for you and/or your family requires persistence and awareness. If something doesn't sound or feel right, chances are it's not. Trust your instincts.

The next step in your journey is to get started.

Dr. Andrew Dine, D.D.S.

www.ingramcontent.com/pod-product-compliance
Lightning Source LLC
Chambersburg PA
CBHW070106210526
45170CB00013B/769